Australian Homoeopathic Home Prescriber

by **Dr Isaac Golden**   Ph.D., D.Hom., N.D., B.Ec.(Hon)

-

Part 1
The Treatment Of Simple Everyday Conditions

4th edition

Australian Homoeopathic Home Prescriber

First published in 1993.
Second Edition   1997, revised 2005.
Third Edition   2007
Fourth Edition   2012

For other books by Dr Isaac Golden, please write to above for a list, or visit the Web site: www.homstudy.net and link to "publications".

Disclaimer:
This book is not intended to replace the services of a qualified practitioner. Any application of the recommendations set forth in the following pages is at the reader's discretion and sole risk.

Prepared for Martin & Pleasance by

Dr Isaac Golden. Ph.D., D.Hom, N.D., B.Ec (Hon).
Principal, Aurum Healing Centre, Gisborne, Victoria.
Principal, Australasian College of Hahnemannian Homoeopathy, Victoria, Australia.
President, Australian Homoeopathic Association (Victorian Branch). 1992-1998.
Deputy Chair, Ethics Committee, National Institute of Integrative Medicine, Australia.

ISBN - 0 - 646 - 15057 – X
ISBN -10: 1481125591
ISBN -13: 978-1481125598
National Library, Canberra. (03) 9245 7397.

CONTENTS

LIST OF EVERYDAY CONDITIONS (CONT)

How to Use This Book

The purpose of this book is to allow you to easily choose Homoeopathic remedies to treat simple everyday or first-aid conditions.

The remedies are all non-toxic and if used sensibly are completely safe. Their sensible use will often prevent the need for chemical drugs or minor surgery.

It is important that if conditions do not respond to the remedies quickly that you seek professional help. At times this will mean seeing a doctor or going to hospital. At other times a qualified natural therapist will be best to see, especially to prevent recurring problems.

So, find your problem in the List of Everyday Conditions just shown, turn to the appropriate page and read the remedy details.

Select the remedy with symptoms that are closest to the symptoms you are experiencing. The conditions *worse from* and *better from* are very important and will often help you to choose between remedies. Even if the symptoms are only similar, the remedy will still help.

It is only possible to show you those remedies which are most likely to help. If the symptoms of your condition really are totally different to the symptoms of the remedies described, you will need to ask a practitioner for help.

How to Use the Remedies

Homoeopathic remedies come as either tiny pilules or drops. Either type of remedy will be effective, so select whichever you prefer.

The number which follows the remedy name is called its **potency**, or strength (e.g. Arnica 30). A potency is suggested with each remedy, but in acute conditions it is OK to use whatever potency you have on hand. The general rule is - the higher the potency, the fewer the number of doses which are needed.

Homoeopathic medicines usually come as drops, or impregnated into little pilules. The latter are very popular with children because they taste great. The usual **dose** is either 5 drops, or 2 pilules of the medicine. Use whichever type of remedy you prefer.

For most acute conditions it is usual to give 2 or 3 doses a day. However, if the symptoms are severe and persistent, you may give doses hourly, or even more often if needed.

It is important to observe the following rules:

1. Don't handle the remedies (i.e. tip pilules onto the lid and then into the mouth, drops can be placed directly under the tongue).
2. Allow the remedy to remain in mouth for 1 minute (preferably under the tongue).
3. Try to give them at least half an hour away from eating,

drinking, brushing the teeth etc.
4. Don't drink coffee or take strongly aromatic food or
drinks.
5. Keep remedies away from strong heat, light or odours.
6. Don't use more than one remedy at a time.

These simple precautions will prevent the remedies from
being antidoted. Remember that we are not using crude,
toxic substances, and our potencies are very sensitive.
This is why they work so well (see page 52 for a brief
introduction to Homoeopathy).

Important Note: If you cannot find the exact problem you
are looking for, try looking up remedies in similar
complaints. For example, if your child has "gastro" you can
look under *Colic, Diarrhoea* and *Food Poisoning*. If you
have sinus congestion, look under *Common Cold,
Influenza* and possibly *Headache.*

ACHES/SPRAINS

Arnica 30 - The first remedy to consider for aching or strained muscles.
Worse from (1) touch, (2) motion, (3) cold damp conditions, or (4) after over exertion.

Aconite 30 or 200 - Sudden onset. Especially useful for a stiff neck. Arms can feel heavy, bruised, numb. Useful for shocked patient.
Worse from (1) a draught of air or cool windy weather, (2) touch.

Dulcamarra 30 - For aching muscles.
Worse from (1) cold damp conditions, (2) night.
Better from (1) movement, (2) warmth.

Rhus Tox. 30 - Strained, sprained, stiff muscles.
Worse from (1) straining or over lifting, especially from stretching high up to reach things, (2) during rest, (3) first movements after rest.
Better from (1) steady motion, (2) warmth.
(note: **Bryonia 30** has the opposite features - better from rest, worse from motion).

Ruta 6 or 30 - For strains of ligaments and tendons after sport or exertion.

NOTE ALSO: Aesculus Hip.6, Ant Tart.30, Colchicum 30, Gelsemium 30, Valerian 30, Veratrum Album 30.

BRUISES

A cold pack or cold water should be quickly applied if possible to help reduce bruising around the injured part.

Arnica 30, 200 - The first remedy for bruises of muscles. Skin has black and blue appearance. Arnica is best taken internally in potency. A lotion or cream of Arnica or Arnica oil may be applied to the area if the skin is not broken. *Worse from* (1) touch, (2) motion, (3) exertion.
Dose - may be given every 10-30 minutes after injury until symptoms improve (which often occurs after a few doses).

Bellis 30 - For bruises of the **breast**. Bruising of deep tissue after surgery.

Hamamelis 6 - Bleeding, with bruised soreness of affected parts. Bruises of **varicose veins.**

Hypericum 6 or 30 - for bruises of parts especially rich in **nerve endings** - esp. fingers and toes.

Ruta 6 or 30 - For bruises of the bones and **tendons**. All parts of the body are painful as if bruised. (Note also **Symphytum 6).**

BURNS/SCALDS

It is essential that any deep-tissue burns be examined in hospital. If very quick relief is not achieved with the remedies (as usually happens with simple burns) seek professional advice.

It is appropriate to take a dose every 10-20 minutes until symptoms lessen.

Cantharis 30 - First remedy for most simple burns. Sunburn. Burns, scalds, with rawness and smarting. Cantharis lotion may also be applied to the area. *Better from* (1) cold applications to burnt area.

Causticum 30 - For painful burn scars. When pain is accompanied by restlessness and blister formation.

Urtica Urens 6 or 30 - For persistent stinging sensations in older burns.

Kali Bichromium 30 - If burns are deep and destroying the skin. Second degree burns leading to or similar to ulcers.

Arsenicum Album 30 - Is often an excellent remedy to treat older burns, especially in hospitalised patients.

Aconite 30 - Can be useful to treat burns where there is great pain and shock.

Carbolic Acid 30 - Useful for acid burns and ulcerated burns.

NOTE ALSO: Hypericum 6, Urtica Urens 30, Aloe Vera externally.

OTHER TREATMENT:

1. Apply cold water to affected areas of first-degree and second-degree burns.
2. A sterile dressing should be applied.
3. Elevate burned areas for severe burns, cover with a sterile dressing (or clean gauze if that is all you have), and seek professional help.
4. **Bach Rescue Remedy**© for shock, plus external applications to 1st and some 2nd degree burns is always helpful.

COLIC IN INFANTS

Colic may lead to a variety of symptoms in infants, such as continual restlessness and crying, broken sleep, poor weight gain etc.

Remedies may be divided into two groups.

1. Child bends forwards or draws knees up.

Colocynthis 6 or 30 - Sharp cutting pains. Cannot keep still. Writhes and twists. Agonising abdominal pains, as if clamped with iron bands. As if internally bruised.
Better from (1) bending double, (2) warmth, (3) pressure.

Chamomilla 30 - Severe, unbearable pain with swelling of the abdomen, crying, writhing and twisting. Cold feet. Often has green "spinach" diarrhoea. Child is **irritable, inconsolable.**
Worse from (1) teething, (2) night.
Better from (1) being carried.

Mag. Phos 6x - Sharp cramping pains. Tired, exhausted patients. Flatulent colic with bloated, full sensation not relieved by belching.
Better from (1) warm applications, (2) rubbing, (3) pressure, (4) after bowel motion.

2. Child straightens up or arches backwards.

Dioscorea Villosa 6 - Severe pains radiate from abdomen. Mouth dry and bitter in the morning.
Worse from (1) pressure on abdomen.
Better from (1) straightening the spine, (2) walking about.

Ipecac 30 - Colic with putrid diarrhoea. Nausea with profuse saliva and a clean tongue.
Better from (1) straightening out.

Nux Vomica 30 - Severe bloating and pressure.
Worse from (1) overfeeding, (2) constipation, (3) pressure.

Belladonna 30 - Distended, hot abdomen. Child is hot and restless, without thirst or sweat.
Worse from (1) jar, (2) pressure, (3) touch.
Better from (1) bending backwards.

NOTE ALSO: China 30, Cina 30 (worms)**, Pulsatilla 30.**

THE COMMON COLD

Obviously, there is no single remedy for the common cold, however the severity of the attack can be significantly reduced with the appropriate remedies. If a patient experiences one cold after another, professional assistance is needed.

Aconite 30 - Often useful in the *first stage* of a cold. The head and face may be burning hot, but the body is cold. Dry short cough which causes a tickling in the back of the throat. Flushed. Great thirst for water. There may be a sore throat, throbbing in the forehead, redness of the eyes and burning of the skin.
Worse from (1) cold wind.

Nux Vomica 30 - Also useful in the *first stage* of a cold; the nose is blocked, or stops at night and runs through the day. There is a frontal headache. Throat is sore and very sensitive to inhaled cold air. The patient is chilly on the least motion or uncovering. Extreme irritability.
Worse from (1) overeating or drinking.

Arsenicum Album 30 - This is a useful remedy in the *second stage* of a cold i.e., watery discharge from the nose sets in causing sore nostrils. Mouth is dry and patient is thirsty (drinks little but often) throat **burns** but is relieved by hot drinks. Great weakness and tiredness, yet the patient is restless. Frequent cold sweats. The skin is cold, but the body feels as though it is **burning** up inside.
Worse at (1) night, especially at midnight.

Pulsatilla 30 - Is useful in the ***third stage*** of a cold. Bland, thick, yellow discharge from the nose or throat, loss of smell and taste, or bitter taste. No thirst and generally poor appetite. Rattling cough with copious, thick, yellow or yellowish-green mucus. Tongue coated with a thick rough white fur, and there may be nausea and vomiting. Ear pains and congestion.
Better from (1) fresh air, (2) consolation.

NOTE ALSO:

Allium Cepa 6 - Sneezing and painless watering eyes. Nose runs like water. Hay fever.
Belladonna 30 - With fever, hacking cough, flushed face, throbbing headache
Gelsemium 30 - Shivers up spine. Fever without thirst. Great fatigue., the patient wants to rest. Flu-like symptoms.
Hepar Sulph 30 - Late stages with thick yellow catarrh. Thick, loose cough.
Euphrasia 6 or 30 - Better lying down at night. Loose cough during day. Profuse watery discharge from the nose. Eyes are red and sore from burning tears.
Mercurius 30 - Profuse sweating, salivation and catarrh. Thick yellow discharge from the nose. Smelly breath. The nose may be ulcerated.
Sanguinaria 6 - Watery catarrh with a tickling dry cough.
Silica 30 - slow onset, slow recovery with sinusitis.
Hydrastis 30 - Stringy, sticky yellow discharge from the nose.
Kali Bich. 30 - Mucus hangs in long strings.

OTHER TREATMENTS:

1. Biochemic
Ferrum Phos 6x - Feverish, sneezing with stuffed nose. Face red or pale.
Nat Mur 6x - Sneezing with thin water discharge from nose.
Kali. Mur. 6x - Mid-stage of cold with heavy, thick clear or white mucus.
Kali Sulph 6x - Thick yellow mucus. Late stage cold. Also **Calc Sulph 6x** for those of solid build.

2. Herbal
Echinacea - Excellent herb for all infections. Has an antibiotic effect.
Garlic - Well known as an effective antibiotic.

3. Other
Vitamin C and **Zinc** - To stimulate immunity.
Diet - Reduce fats, dairy and refined foods.

CONCUSSION

Common sense must be used whenever there are any head injuries, and medical attention must be sought unless the patient makes a rapid and complete recovery. Watch for severe headaches, blurred vision, vomiting, extreme drowsiness or dizziness.

Arnica 30 or 200: - for immediate first aid, especially when there is visible bruising.
Dose: Can be given every 10-30 minutes in serious acute cases. Otherwise 3 times daily.

Nat Sulph 200 - In high potency is the best treatment for the remaining effects of past concussion, or to follow Arnica in recent concussion if the patient is not fully recovered. Give doses twice a week.

NOTE ALSO:

Cicuta 30 - when there are muscle twitching or convulsions.
Helleborus 30 - for a persistent overwhelming headache.
Kali Phos 6x or 30 - for persistent insomnia after concussion.
Bach Rescue Remedy© - for initial shock.

CONSTIPATION

Patients either want to pass a motion but cannot, or are constipated without urging or discomfort.

Type 1 - Desires to pass a motion.

Nux Vomica 30 - For thin, irritable, critical people. **Ineffectual urging**. Frequent desire, but only very little passes. Rectum never feels empty even after a motion. Business people who rush.
Worse from (1) overeating of rich foods or (2) overuse of laxatives, alcohol or coffee.

Magnesia Muriatica 30 - Stool like sheep's dung and difficult OR thin and brown with burning pains. Pain in region of liver. Stools crumble as if burnt.

Nitricum Acidum 30 - Hard, scanty stool. Painful in passing (can last for hours). Severe burning in rectum or great itching. Sensation of sticks in the rectum. Patient loves salts and fats.

Type 2 - No desire to pass a motion.

Alumina 30 - No urging for days, yet has a soft stool which is difficult to pass. May have mucus with stool. Patient is often thin, spare, wrinkled, cold sensitive, dry mouth. Can help children who have been fed on formulas.

Opium 30 - Absence of desire. Stools are round, hard, dry balls. Poor appetite with intense thirst.

Bryonia Alba 30 - Often no urge for many days without discomfort. Stools are often large, hard, dry, look burned and are painful. Can occur with a splitting headache. *Worse from* (1) warm weather.

Hydrastis Canadensis 30 - No desire for stool. Constipation alternating with looseness of the bowels. With dull headache, foul tongue, piles. *Worse after* (1) abuse of purgatives.

NOTE ALSO: **Calc. Carb.30** (patient feels better when constipated), **Lycopodium 30** (rumbling in bowel), **China 30, Graphites 30, Silica 30** (large, hard, difficult motion).

FLATULENCE: This may be the result from a variety of conditions. If you examine remedies under Diarrhoea, Colic, Constipation and Food Poisoning you should find a remedy to help. Note in particular **Chamomilla 30, Lycopodium 30** and **Carbo Veg 30**.

COUGH/CROUP

There are hundreds of remedies which will help to relieve various types of cough. You may need a practitioner's help if you cannot find a remedy with similar symptoms. Recurring coughs need professional attention.

Hyoscyamus 30 - Cough forces patient to sit up.
Worse from (1) lying down (comes on quickly).
Better from (1) sitting up.

Ant. Tart. 30 - Loose, choking, **rattling**, wheezing. Thick, difficult expectoration. Face turns blue.
Worse from (1) cold damp weather, (2) night.
Better from (1) sitting up.

Drosera 30 - Dry barking cough. Tickling, wheezing. Often causes retching. Face purple. Holds chest with hands while coughing.
Worse from (1) lying down, (2) night.

NOTE ALSO:
Dry Cough - **Aconite 30, Bryonia, Rumex 30, Spongia 30.**

Loose Cough - **Ipecac 30, Hepar Sulph 30, Phosphorus 30, Pulsatilla 30.**

Spasmodic Cough - **Coccus Cacti 30, Cuprum Met 30.**

CROUP

The three remedies given in the order shown have proven to be very effective in most cases of Croup.

1. **Aconite 200** - First stage only. Dry cough. Sudden onset. Hot head, cold extremities.
Worse from (1) exposure to (cold) wind.

2. **Hepar Sulph 200** - Second stage. Loose thick cough. Barking. Feels as if a needle or splinters in throat.
Worse from (1) cold air, (2) sunset, sunrise.
Better from (1) warm moist air (e.g. a vaporiser, steam from a shower etc.).

3. **Spongia 200** - Third stage. Dry, noisy, barking cough. Wheezing with constriction.
Worse from (1) breathing in, (2) cold drinks.
Better from (1) bending forwards.

Begin with a dose of 1. Repeat within two hours then, if necessary, move to 2 for two doses, and then 3.

CUTS AND WOUNDS

Medical attention must be sought if the wound is serious or if bleeding persists.

Calendula tincture or cream - Antiseptic for simple cuts, abrasions and lacerated wounds. Promotes healthy granulations and rapid healing.

Staphysagria 30 - For clean-cut wounds, glass etc. Pains are excruciating, rending and tearing, causing great agony Surgery especially about the abdomen when colic follows. **Anger.**

Ledum 30 - For puncture wounds. Prevents sepsis. The premier anti-tetanus remedy.

Comfrey tincture or cream - Apply **only** when all possibility of infection ceases. It will speed up healing of damaged skin.

Hypericum 30, tincture or cream - useful antiseptic and anti-tetanus. Often combined with **Calendula** to make **Hypercal cream** which is excellent for all cuts and wounds.

NOTE ALSO: for scars consider **Thiosinamine 6** and **Graphites 6 or 30** (keloid).

CYSTITIS/BLADDER INFLAMMATION

Symptoms must not be allowed to develop as a kidney infection may follow. Drink plenty of water, eat lots of vegetables, avoid acid foods. Careful personal hygiene is essential.

Cantharis 6 or 30 - Constant desire to urinate, but only a few drops pass. Burning and stinging before, during and after urination.

Berberis 6 or 30 - Burning and cutting pains during and after urination. Constant desire.

Apis 6 - Constant desire. Increased amount of urine. Sharp stinging pains on urination.

Staphysagria 6 or 30 - Burning between urination.
Worse from (1) intercourse.
Better from (1) passing urine.

Equisetum 6 - Frequent urination. Bed wetting in children.
Worse (1) during and after urination.

Note also: Terebinthina 30, Belladonna 30, Causticum 30, Golden Seal tincture as a wash.

NOTE: Cystitis is often caused by a proliferation of the Candida Albicans organism. See a practitioner to identify and remove this possible cause.

DIARRHOEA

If Diarrhoea persists, especially in young children, medical advice must be sought to ensure the patient does not become dehydrated.

Arsenicum Album 30 - With vomiting. Diarrhoea in small quantities with violent, **burning** pains in abdomen. Offensive. Patient is emotionally restless but physically weak. Pale face, cold body, dry tongue. Stool usually dark, scanty, watery or mucus, sometimes bloody,
Worse after (1) eating, (2) drinking,
(3) midnight.
Better from (1) warm applications, (2) drinks.

Dulcamara 30 - Stool is watery without much pain.
Worse from (1) **cold and damp**, (2) at night.

Rheum 30 - For sour smelling stools. Thin, slimy fermented diarrhoea, common to small children. **Sour** smell proceeding from the child, which washing will not remove. Diarrhoea from acidity of the stomach. Crying, both before and after a stool. Ineffectual urging both after and before a stool.

Bryonia 30 -   Dry mouth, with thirst for large quantities of water at long intervals, and a desire to lie down and remain quiet.
Worse from (1) sour fruit, (2) in warmer weather

Pulsatilla 30 - Stools usually green, variable. Much rumbling and gas. Tongue coated white. Bitter taste and dryness in the mouth without thirst. Chilliness. Can feel as though she has overeaten even after a light meal.
Worse from (1) fats, rich foods, ice cream, fruits, (2) at night with gnawing pains in stomach.
Better from (1) fresh air.

Phosphorus 30 - Especially useful for chronic forms of diarrhoea, white watery discharge passing out with great force as from a pipe. Watery stool with lumps of white mucus, or little grains like rice or sago.
Worse from (1) warm food, (2) after eating.
Better after (2) cold food.

Podophyllum 6 or 30 - Watery **yellow** stools in the morning, with a sense of weakness in the rectum. Offensive odour.

NOTE ALSO: Colocynthis 6, Chamomilla 30, Sulphur 6, Veratrum Album 30.

EARACHE

Care must be taken to ensure that the eardrum is not ruptured, or that secondary infections do not develop. These are unlikely if the symptoms clear quickly.

Mullein oil or tincture - Use the warm oil or tincture externally in the ear to provide immediate 1st aid relief. (Garlic oil and Hypericum oil also are helpful to relieve the pain). Use internal remedies as well as the Mullein.

Aconite 30 - Recent inflammation. External ear red, hot, painful, Patient is thirsty.
Worse from (1) cold, (2) draught of air or wind, (3) evening, (4) swallowing.
Better from (1) warm applications, (2) eating.

Belladonna 30 - Sudden onset of digging, boring, violent pains. Face is red, congested, hot with swelling of ear with pus formation. Shooting **throbbing** pains. Extend to the throat. Pain causes screaming and delirium. Thirstless.

Hepar Sulph 30 - Inflammation. When pus is forming, before discharge. Ear feels bruised and sore. Whizzing, throbbing sounds in ear.
Worse from (1) slightest touch, (2) any exposure to cold air.

Pulsatilla 6 or 30 - Sticking and tearing pains in and behind the ears. Swelling and feeling as if ears were closed. May be a profuse, thick, yellow/green discharge. Difficult hearing. Red external ear. **6c** will "drain" the eustachian tubes.
Worse from (1) at night, (2) dairy or fatty foods.
Better from (1) cold applications.

Chamomilla 30 - Earache from cold or suppressed perspiration. Stabbing, tearing pains in the ears. Extreme sensitiveness and irritability. Child is angry and in great pain.
Worse from (1) stooping, (2) night, (3) warmth, (4) teething.
Better from (1) being carried.

Sulphur 30 - If the pain returns frequently. Ear is red and itchy. Deafness, with noises in the ear.
Worse (1) in evening, before midnight, (2) left.

Rhus. Tox. 30 -. Inflammation of middle ear with thick yellow discharge. Itching and crawling as if something alive inside.
Worse from (1) getting wet in rain, (2) bathing in the river, (3) suppressed perspiration.

NOTE ALSO: Apis 6 or 30, Kali. Mur. 6x, Mercurius 30.

EYES - INFLAMMATION AND DISCHARGES

Aconite 30 - For acute conjunctivitis. Profuse discharge with swelling of lids and excessive pain. Sudden onset.
Worse (1) at night, (2) warm room, (3) wind.
Better in (1) the open air.

Arnica 30 - For inflammation from external injuries. Black eye.

Belladonna 30 - Dry infected eyes, total absence of tears. Symptoms are intense and violent. Thickened red lids. Dilated pupils.
Worse from (1) light.

Arsenicum Album 30 - Red, painful, **burning** inflammation inside eyelids. Eyes can scarcely be opened. Acrid, **burning discharge**.
Worse (1) after midnight.
Better from (1) warm applications.

Mercurius Solubilis 30 - Eyes swollen, difficult to open. Pain is cutting with edges ulcerated and scabs on the outside. Often follows **Belladonna** well. Discharge of pus.

Hepar Sulph 30 - Is useful if **Merc Sol** does not produce a favourable change. Discharge of pus.
Worse from (1) touch, (2) air, (3) cold winds.

Euphrasia 6 or 30 - Catarrhal conjunctivitis. Burning and swelling of lids. Thick discharge. Eyes water all the time. The tincture or tea can be used as an eyewash.
Worse in (1) evening, (2) indoors, (3) warmth.
Better from (1) open air, (2) dark.

Gelsemium 30 - Soreness of the eyeballs. Pain in the eyeballs. Double vision. Giddiness. Often accompanies the flu.

Sulphur 30 - Use after Aconite or Arnica in cases where the sensation of smarting still continues. Redness and heat. Sharp, sticking pains. Itching of lids.

Pulsatilla 6 or 30 - Discharge is thick, yellow, bland, profuse. Lids glued together especially on waking. Caused by rubbing eyes.
Better from (1) open air.

Silica 30 - Inflammation persisting after injury from a foreign body.

NOTE ALSO: Allium Cepa. 6, Arg. Nit. 30, Kali Hydr. 30, Symphytum 6.

FEVER

Fever is a natural response which, if managed well, can be beneficial to the patient. The onset of perspiration will often resolve the fever, but do not overdress or cover the patient to try to force this. Cool bathing and frequent drinks will help to lower the temperature.

Temperatures:
Normal resting temperature - 37°C (98.6°F).
Low grade fever - 37.5 - 38.2°C (99.5 - 101°F).
High grade fever - above 38.2°C (101°F).

1. Sudden onset fevers.

Aconite 30 or 200 - Sudden onset, restless, fearful. Hot head, cold hands and feet. Dry, burning skin. Anxiety and fear.
Worse from (1) cold air, (2) wind, (3) night.

Belladonna 30 - Violent onset. Face dark red, flushed. Eyes glazed, watery. Delirious. **Heat without sweat or thirst**. Cold extremities. With throat symptoms and headache. Burning, dry skin.

2. Steady onset fevers.

Ferrum Phos 6x - useful support in all cases, especially slow building fever. Face red. Low grade fever with sweating.

Gelsemium 30 - Trembling. **Chills** up spine. Wants to lie still. **Weakness**. Thirstless. Heavy aching feeling. Flu-type symptoms.

3. Other fevers.

Nux Vomica 30 - Patient is irritable, restless.
Worse from (1) exposure to cold, (2) excessive use of coffee, tobacco, heavy spiced foods or alcohol, (3) overheating.

Rhus Tox. 30 - Patient is restless and must move constantly.
Worse from (1) getting wet in the rain, (2) heavy perspiration, (rest).

Bryonia 30 - Patient wants to lie still and quiet. Body aches all over. Dry mouth with thirst.
Worse from (1) warm summer weather, (2) movement, (3) coughing.
Better from (1) rest, (2) cool drinks.

Arsenicum Album 30 - Restless, agitated but weak. Alternating hot and cold. Desires frequent small amounts of water.
Worse (1) after midnight.
Better from (2) warmth.

FOOD POISONING

The following remedies are for mild cases. Seek assistance if symptoms do not respond quickly.

Arsenicum Album 30 - With nausea and vomiting. **Burning** in the stomach. **Restlessness**. Despairing. Intense thirst - drinks little but often. Craves ice water which is vomited (Phos.). Violent abdominal pains. Rolls about in anguish.
Worse after (1) spoiled food, especially meat and watery fruit.

Carbo Vegetablis 6 or 30 - Patient is **lifeless**. Cold body and breath (but hot head). Weak pulse, quick breathing - **needs air** (to be fanned). Skin blue. Flatulent. Loud belching. Burning in stomach. Vomiting of blood.

Nux Vomica 30 - Patient is restless and **irritable**. Belching of sour fluid into mouth. Nausea and vomiting with much retching.
Worse from (1) abuse of food and/or alcohol.

NOTE ALSO: The **Giardia Nosode M** is often excellent as both primary treatment and a preventative.

FRIGHT/SHOCK

Bach Rescue RemedyR - Invaluable acute emergency remedy for all trauma/shock. Give 2 drops of stock strength every few minutes until the patient becomes calm.

Aconite 30 or 200 - Fright with collapse or fever. Patient agitated and restless. Fear of death. Sudden onset.

Veratrum Album 30 - Cold sweat on forehead and body. Surgical shock. Is a heart stimulant. **Note** also **Carbo Veg. 30** (difficult breathing, and arrested circulation, must have air).

Arnica 30 - After mental strain, shock, physical trauma. Fear of being touched. Nausea, pain.

Opium 30 - With coma or complete inactivity. Extremities and face are bluish or a livid colour. Loud breathing. OR convulsions and trembling.

Camphor 30 - Use if **Opium 30** fails. Hands and feet cold and trembling. Sudden prostration.

Ignatia 30 - Hysteria. Loss of control. Insomnia *Worse from* (1) grief, (2) disappointed love.

NOTE ALSO: Coffea 30, Gelsemium 30, Nat. Mur. 30, Phos. Acid. 30.

GOUT

Diet must be changed to eliminate foods rich in purines, e.g. sardines, anchovies, shellfish, offal. Try to eliminate alcohol, caffeine and smoking.

Colchicum 6 or 30 - First remedy in many cases. Dejected, weak, nauseous. Shooting and tearing pain in muscles and joints, which are red, hot, swollen and stiff, *Worse from* (1) touch, (2) movement, (3) night.

Pulsatilla 30 - Useful when gout is in the forming stage. Pain moves from joint to joint. Joints swollen, red and oedematous.
Worse from (1) allowing affected limbs to hang down.
Better from (1) cold applications.

Ledum Palustre 30 - Subacute gout. Affected parts are purple and puffy. Pains particularly in small joints.
The **patient** is *worse from* (1) cold air.
The **affected part** is *better from* (1) cold air and bathing.

Lycopodium 30 - When one foot is hot and the other is cold. Deep acting remedy.
Better from (1) movement, (2) after midnight.

NOTE ALSO: Apis, Uric Acid.

HEADACHES

If headaches recur, ask a practitioner to find and remove the cause. The few remedies listed below are a starting point only, as hundreds are available.

Bryonia 30 - Frequently used remedy. Dry mouth. Bursting pain, especially in the forehead.
Worse from (1) movement, (2) stooping, (3) heat.
Better from (1) rest - wants to lie quiet and still, (2) a dark room, (3) pressure.

Nux Vomica 30 - Patient is irritable. Very cold. Piercing frontal pain. Tension in neck pain.
Worse from (1) alcohol, stimulants, rich food,
(2) anger, (3) excessive mental stress or worry,
(4) light, (5) insomnia.

Glonoine 30 - Sudden throbbing, bursting, hammering pain.
Worse from (1) exposure to **sun**, (2) high blood pressure.

Gelsemium 30 - Feels like a band around head. Dull heavy pain. Shivering up the spine. Trembling.
Worse from (1) emotional shock, (2) influenza.
Better from (1) pressure, (2) urination.

NOTE ALSO: Ruta 30 (eyestrain), **Belladonna 30** (fever with violent throbbing, dilated pupils), **Cocculus 30** (travel), **Arnica 30** (injury, exertion).

HEARTBURN / INDIGESTION

Nat Phos 6x - Excellent first-aid remedy for simple acidity. Repeat every 5 minutes if needed.

Nux Vomica 30 - With flatulence, nausea and vomiting. **Irritable**. Sour, bitter belching.
Worse from (1) overeating, (2) alcohol, (3) morning.

Capsicum 6 or 30 - Burning sensation in stomach and the length of the bowel. Much thirst, but drinking causes shuddering.

Pulsatilla 30 - Dislikes warm food, drink. Craves acids, or what disagrees. Thirstless. Taste of food remains. Feels like a stone in the stomach.
Worse from (1) rich foods, fats, ices, eggs.

Arg. Nit. 30 - For simple heartburn. **Craves sugar** which aggravates. Desires cheese. Eating relieves nausea but makes the stomach worse. Sour foods relieve nausea.

NOTE ALSO: **Arsenicum Album 30, Carbo. Veg. 6 or 30, Lycopodium 30, Mancinella 30, Phosphorous 6, Sulphur 6 or 30.**

HOARSENESS

Arnica 30 - *Worse from* (1) severe overuse, e.g. shouting, screaming, singing.

Phosphorus 6 or 30 - Larynx very painful. Pain or violent tickling in larynx while speaking. Cough from tickling in throat.
Worse (1) in evening, (2) cold air.

Causticum 6 or 30 - Scraping, **burning,** rawness. Difficult swallowing. Difficulty in removing mucus. Desires cold drinks.
Worse from (1) excessive use, (2) morning.

Rhus Tox 30 - Hoarseness at beginning of speaking or singing, better from continued use, then worse again at the end. (**Bryonia 30** is better from rest, worse from use of voice).

Arum.Triph.30 - Pitch of voice varies. Difficult to control.
Worse from (1) singing and talking.
Better from (1) rest.

NOTE ALSO: Aconite 30, Ant. Crud. 30, Argentum Met. 30, Argentum Nit. 30, Drosera 30, Hepar Sulph. 6, Spongia 30.

INFLUENZA

Care must be taken to ensure the condition does not progress to secondary infections. Seek help from a practitioner if in doubt. A practitioner will also be able to help with preventative treatment.

Eupatorium Perf. 30 - Deep seated, violent, aching **bone pains**, especially in the back, wrists and ankles. Eye balls sore on turning. Vomiting and debility. The patient is restless, chilly, nauseated. Thirstless, or thirst for cold drinks.

Gelsemium 30 - Severe bodily pain with great **weakness**. The patient wants to lie perfectly still. Trembling from weakness with the least exertion. Fever with no thirst. The tongue trembles when producing it. Dry cough with sore chest, gives burning larynx and chest. Chills up spine. *Worse from* (1) damp weather.

Nux Vomica 30 - After drinking, immediately shivering and chilliness. Chilliness on the least movement. On the slightest exposure to the open air, shivering and chilliness for an hour. Dreads to go into open air. He cannot get warm. Attack, as of fever. Shivering and drawing in the limbs. Violent cough (wants to eat during the cough).

Arsenicum Album 30 - Copious discharge from the nose. Restlessness with great weakness and prostration. Difficult breathing. Scanty, frothy expectoration. Shortness of breath with **restlessness**. **Burning** or coldness in chest.

Better from (1) sitting up.

Bryonia 30 - Severe pain in the whole of the body, wanting to lie quiet, and still. Mouth and throat dry with great thirst. Headache and severe constipation. Cough dry, hard, painful.
Worse from (1) least motion, (2) deep breathing.

Oscillococcinum 200 - This remedy is used internationally as a preventative, as well as treatment for the common symptoms of Influenza.

NOTE ALSO:
1st stage - **Aconite 30, Belladonna 30 (fast onset), Ferrum Phos 6x. (slow onset).**
2nd stage - **Gelsemium 30, Eup. Perf. 30, Bryonia 30.**

NOTE ALSO: Baptisia 30, Camphor 30, Pyrogen 30, Rhus Tox. 30, Veratrum Album 30.

INSECT BITES

Give the patient **Bach Rescue Remedy**® if they are distressed. Often cold water or ice pack will help.

Ledum 30 - For mosquito bites or stings from other small insects. Affected parts are purple, puffy, cold.
Worse from (1) jarring motion, (2) warmth to part.

Apis 6 or 30 - For bee, hornet and wasp stings. Rosy red shiny **swelling** of the part which **burns or stings** like hot needles. Exhausted yet restless.
Worse from (1) heat or hot applications, (2) touch.

Carbolicum Acidum 30 - For poisonous spider, scorpion and snake bites. Burning, itching vesicles which tend to ulcerate. Malignant and septic conditions after bites. Exhaustion. Unsteadiness.

Lachesis 30 - For spider, scorpion and snake bites Part becomes dull red or blue. Thin dark bleeding.
Worse from (1) heat in general.
Better from (1) open air.

Formica Rufa 30 - Ant bites. Sudden rheumatic or gouty pains. Profuse sweat without relief. Cold.

Urtica Urens 30 - Itchy, blotchy - like nettle rash.

NOTE ALSO: Staphysagria 30 (with anger, better warmth), **Hypericum 30** (bites on fingers and toes).

INSOMNIA

Treat the cause where possible rather than sedate.

Aconite 30 - Intense anxiety, fear. Nightmares.
Worse from (1) fear, (2) fright, (3) anxiety.

Nux Vomica 30 - With poor digestion. Awakes too early, cannot go to sleep again after waking.
Worse from (1) excessive coffee, tea, alcohol, (2) mental overwork at night, (3) rush of ideas.

Sulphur 30 - Drowsy all day and sleepless at night. Difficult to get back to sleep. Catnaps. Vivid dreams.
Worse from (1) nervous excitement, (2) skin itch, (3) external heat, esp. in bed, (4) slight noise.

Opium 30 - Patient sleepy but cannot sleep. **For the elderly**. Disturbed by ordinary noises.

Phosphorous 30 - Short naps, frequent wakening. In morning feels as though he has not slept.
Worse from (1) mental overwork and anxiety.

Ignatia 30 - Every sound awakens. Jerking of limbs on going to sleep. Horrid dreams.
Worse from (1) grief, (2) worry, (3) fright, (4) disappointed love (Nat Mur in chronic cases).

Coffea 30 - Cannot stop thinking, especially after happy news.

NAUSEA/VOMITING

If nausea or vomiting persists, consult a practitioner to investigate the cause. Watch for dehydration with constant vomiting.

Nat Sulph 6x - the best simple first-aid remedy for nausea.
Dose - one tablet every 10 minutes as needed.

Ipecac 6 or 30 - Copious vomiting with **persistent nausea** even after vomiting. Intense nausea with sweating. Griping pain in intestines. Tongue is clean, with profuse saliva.
Worse from (1) least drink.

Antimonium Crud. 6 or 30 - Nausea. Thickly coated white tongue. Eructations. Loss of appetite. Irritable and complaining. Vomits soon after eating or drinking.
Worse from (1) overeating, (2) poor diet.

Arsenicum Album 30 - Burning in stomach and throat. **Weakness**. Purging. coldness of the hands and feet. Vomiting with diarrhoea. Acid vomiting.
Worse from (1) spoiled food, (2) bad meat, (3) watery fruit, (4) after midnight.

Pulsatilla 30 - Thirstless. Excessive mucus.
Worse from (1) rich, fatty foods, (2) during pregnancy.
Better in (1) open air.

Nux Vomica 30 - The best hangover remedy. Heartburn.

Belching. Bloated heavy feeling in stomach.
Worse from (1) overeating or drinking, (2) morning.

Cocculus 30 - For travel nausea and sickness.

Iris 30 - For nausea and vomiting accompanying a migraine.

Aethusa 30 - For infants who cannot digest milk without vomiting.

Phosphorous 30 - Great thirst for cold water, which is vomited as soon as it becomes warm in the stomach.

NOTE ALSO: **Colocynthis 6 or 30, Veratrum Album 30.**

NETTLE RASH/URTICARIA

Apis 6 or 30 - Swelling, heat, redness of affected part, especially eyelids and lips.
Worse from (1) heat of any kind.

Nux Vomica 30 - When there are gastric upsets with constipation. Scratching and itching.
Worse from (1) indulgence in alcohol.

Rhus Tox. 30 - Little blisters which burn and itch. Area can be stiff.

Urtica Urens 6 - Blotches with violent itching.
Worse from (1) water, (2) cold moist air, (3) touch.

Belladonna 30 - When the eruption is attended by violent headache, hot and red face. The children cry a lot. Rubbing eases the itching.

Sulphur 6 or 30 - Dry, burning, itching rash.
Worse from (1) bathing, (2) wool, (3) heat.

NOTE ALSO: Aconite 30, Bryonia 30, Dulcamarra 30, Pulsatilla 30, Urtica Urens cream.

NOSE BLEEDS

Homoeopathy has an ability to cure the tendency to recurring bleeding, as well as being helpful in sudden bleeding. Seek help if bleeding is not rapidly reduced.

Millefolium 30 - Good first aid in simple nose bleeds.

Phosphorous 30 - Recurring nose bleeds in slender, sensitive people. Profuse, bright blood.
Following injury.

Ferrum Phos 6x - No obvious cause. Recurring.
Good for children during fevers.

Aconite 30 - Sudden profuse bleeding, often during fever or headache. With fear.

Arnica 30 - Following injury. Blowing nose too much.

Hamamelis 6 - When there are problems with veins elsewhere, e.g. varicose veins, haemorrhoids.

PILES/HAEMORRHOIDS

1. Bleeding Haemorrhoids.

Hamamelis Virginica 6 - Haemorrhoids bleeding profusely, with soreness like a bruise.

Aloe 6 or 30 - Very sore, tender, protruding. Bleeding. Burning sensation.
Better from (1) cold water application.

Muriaticum Acidum 30 - Haemorrhoids most sensitive to all touch; even sheet of toilet paper is painful.

2. Non-Bleeding Haemorrhoids

Aesculus Hipp. 6 - Blind haemorrhoids, with sharp shooting pains up the back. Prolapse of rectum. Dry, burning, itching rectum.

Paeonia 30 - Much pain during and after a bowel action, and often with a fissure.
Worse (1) during and after bowel motion.

Sulphur 6 or 30 - Constipation with ineffectual urging, or loose motion in the early morning. **Itching** anus. Violent shooting pain in back. Headache.
Worse from (1) bathing.

NOTE ALSO: Arnica 30 (childbirth), **Nit. Acid 30**

SKIN PROBLEMS

Apart from contact dermatitis, most skin conditions arise from internal problems which must be treated. Diet is often a factor. Delay giving further doses if the skin gets worse following a remedy.

Psorinum 30 - Intolerable itching. Dry, dirty looking skin. Appears unwashed even if clean. Bad smell.
Worse from (1) winter, (2) cold.

Sulphur 6 or 30 - Dry, red rash. Itching, burning.
Worse from (1) heat of bed, (2) warm bathing.

Hepar Sulph 30 - Suppurating, festering sores. Boils. Abscesses.

Silica 6x or 30 - Injuries won't heal. Cracks. Bed sores. Abscesses. Profuse offensive sweat.

Mezereum 30 - Violent itch with burning. May be scabby. School sores. Herpes. Shingles.
Worse from (1) scratching, (2) heat of bed.

NOTE ALSO: Petroleum 6 or 30 (dark, cracked skin), **Graphites 6 or 30** (cracks, yellow sticky discharge). **See also: *Nettle Rash*.**

SUNBURN

Cantharis 6 or 30 - Sunburn with rawness and smarting, followed by undue inflammation.
Better from (1) cold applications.

Hypericum 6 - Burned area may be covered with Hypericum lotion.

**Note also: Bufo Rana 6, Kali Carbonicum 30.
Aloe Vera gel.**

SUNSTROKE

Glonoine 30 - With **throbbing** headache. Face flushed and sweating.

Belladonna 30 - **Throbbing** headache. Hot dry skin without thirst. Delirium. Dilated pupils.

Ant. Crud. 30 - *Worse from* (1) exertion in the sun.

Gelsemium 30 - Giddiness as if the patient has been drinking.

NOTE ALSO: Aconite 30, Cuprum Metallicum 30.

TEETHING PROBLEMS

Chamomilla 30 - Often the first remedy to consider. Unbearable pain. The child is fretful and angry. Inconsolable. One cheek is red, one pale. Diarrhoea like chopped up spinach.
Better from (1) **being carried.**

Belladonna 30 - Convulsions. Child is irritable, flushed, restless and delirious.

Calcarea Carbonicum 30 - Teething is slow in fat, fair, sweaty children (**Calc. Phos. 30** for thinner children with similar symptoms). Follows Chamomilla or Belladonna well.

Cina 30 - Given in particular to children who wet the bed at night,and grind their teeth during sleep and other times.
Worse from - worm infestations.

Mercurius 30 - Excessive sweat and **saliva.** Red gums. Green stools with straining.

Borax 30 - Teething with mouth ulcers.
Worse from (1) downward motion, e.g. while being placed in a cot.

NOTE ALSO: **Silica 30, Sulphur 30.**

THROAT INFLAMMATION/TONSILLITIS

Mercury 30 - Profuse **saliva.** Perspiration. Burning pain goes into ears. Patient alternates between being too hot or too cold. Bad breath.
Worse from (1) swallowing.

Aconite 30 - Sudden onset in feverish conditions. Craves cold drinks.
Worse from (1) cold wind.

Phytolacca 6 - Will clear the lymphatic system after some months of regular use, and help prevent recurring tonsillitis. Throat dark red, **swollen,** painful.
Worse from (1) swallowing.

Hepar Sulph 6 or 30 - Glands swollen and sensitive. Pain like a splinter in throat. Ulceration and yellow pus.
Worse from (1) cold air, (2) draughts, (3) uncovering.

NOTE ALSO: Merc. Iod. Flavus (right sided), **Merc. Iod. Ruber** (left sided), **Lac Caninum** (alternating sides). **Lachesis 30, Calc Carb 30, Sulphur 30**.

THRUSH/MOUTH ULCERS

Borax 30 - Established ulcers. Small red vesicles become ulcers. Child cries when nursing. Dread of downward motion. Very painful with grey base. Pain *worse from* (1) touch, (2) acid, salty food.

Mercury 30 - Profuse **saliva**. Metallic taste with thirst plus slimy diarrhoea. Shallow burning ulcers. Tongue soft, swollen. Teeth indented, yellow. Neck glands swollen and painful.

Natrum Mur. 30 - With hepatic vesicles (blisters) on the lips. Clear vesicles. Ulcers like pearls.

Nitric Acid 30 - Irregular edges which bleed. Stinging, sticking pain. Infants who vomit milk.

Capsicum 6 or 30 - Hot sensations in the mouth worse from cold water. Bad smell from mouth.

Hydrastis 6 or 30 - Tongue swollen. Cold sores on lower lips. Ulcers on inside of lower lip. Thick sticky saliva. Use the tincture externally both for oral and vaginal ulceration.

NOTE ALSO: **Arsenicum 30, Kali Chloricum 30, Rhus. Tox. 30.**
Externally **- Propolis, Golden Seal tincture, Tea Tree oil.**

TRAVEL SICKNESS

Borax 30 - *Worse from* downward movement, e.g. aircraft or lifts.

Cocculus 6 or 30 - Often used remedy - with vertigo and emptiness in the head. Metallic taste in the mouth with increased saliva (**Mercury**).
Worse from (1) the thought, sight, smell of food.
Better from (1) warmth.

Petroleum 6 or 30 - Nausea and eructations of wind from the stomach. **Saliva**. Empty feeling. Vomiting and giddiness worse from noise. Pain in the neck and the occiput.
Better from (1) eating, (2) closing eyes.

Tabacum 6 or 30 - With cold sweat and weakness. Headache like a band around the head. Very pale face. Fainting.
Worse from (1) smell of smoke.
Better from (1) the cold.

NOTE ALSO:
Anxiety before the journey: **Argent. Nit. 30.**, **Gelsemium 30, Ignatia 30, Lycopodium 30.**
Overexcitement before the journey: **Coffea Cruda 6.**

A Homoeopathic First Aid Kit

One problem in selecting a list of remedies to include in a First Aid Kit is that there are so many available. The Following list would provide an excellent starting Kit.

Aconite 30	Euphrasia 6
Arnica 30	Gelsemium 30
Arsenicum Album 30	Ipecac. 30
Acid. Phos. 30	Ledum 30
Belladonna 30	Mercurius 30
Bryonia 30	Nux Vomica 30
Carbo Veg. 30	Phosphorous 30
Cantharis 30	Pulsatilla 30
Chamomilla 30	Rhus Tox. 30
Colocynthis 6	Rescue Remedy
Arnica Cream or Lotion	Burn Cream
Calendula Cream	Hypercal Cream
or Lotion.	Tea Tree Cream

A Kit similar to this is available from Martin & Pleasance, 7 Rocklea Drive, Port Melbourne VIC 3207. Phone (03) 9427 7422.

Note that this list is a starting point only, and many parents will want to add to their basic Kit once they become more experienced with different remedies and find other remedies which they need.

A Brief Explanation of Homoeopathy

Homoeopathy has been used for 200 years in most countries around the world. It is used extensively by doctors, as well as natural therapists.

It is unfortunate that in Australia the local medical community has resisted its widespread use, although this is sure to change as they are brought up to date with their medical colleagues overseas.

Homoeopathy was founded by a German doctor, Dr Samuel Hahnemann, who was a brilliant physician and pharmacist. Because of his fluency in seven languages he was able to read healing texts from all communities and all ages.

He was the first physician to make full practical use of a Law of Nature known to ancient healers such as Hippocrates. This was the **Law of Similars** which states that a substance which is capable of causing a group of symptoms in a healthy person is capable of removing a group of **similar** symptoms in an unwell person.

Dr Hahnemann realised the value of this Law when he was translating a book of medicines from English into German. He disagreed with the author's description of the effects of overdoses of Peruvian Bark, a Herb which was used in the treatment of Malarial fevers.

Dr Hahnemann, being a true scientist, experimented by

taking small doses of the Bark and found that he developed a fever **which was very similar to a Malarial fever.** The fever stopped when he stopped taking the Bark. He took some more, and the fever started again. It stopped soon after he stopped taking the Bark.

This was a practical example of the Law of Similars, i.e. the Bark was capable of producing in a healthy person a fever **similar** to what it could cure in an unwell person.

Over the last 200 years, Homoeopaths have **"proved"** thousands of substances. Unlike drug testing, we test our medicines on healthy volunteers who report the resulting symptoms, which are then very carefully and systematically compiled into a description of what symptoms the substance can remove in unwell patients. It **is** very scientific.

This is why, when you come to choose a medicine to use from the ones given in the book, that you select the medicine whose symptoms are **the most similar** to the symptoms of your patient. It is then prescribed in the minimum dose necessary to produce a healing response.

Resource Page/Other Reading

Some good introductory books:
Isaac Golden – *AHHP Part 2 – A Simple Materia Media of Common Remedies with Repertory*.
Isaac Golden – *AHHP Part 3 – A Simple Introduction to Homoeopathic Medicine*.
George Vithoulkas - *Homoeopathy: Medicine of the New Man*.
S & R Gibson - *Homoeopathy for Everyone*.
Dr M.T. Santwani - *Common Ailments of Children and their Homoeopathic Management*.
Martin & Pleasance - *Handbook of the Biochemic Tissue Salts*.

Homoeopathic correspondence courses by the Australasian College of Hahnemannian Homoeopathy:
1. *An Introductory Course in Natural Medicine*. Introduces Mum's and Dad's to how prescribe a range of natural remedies, including homoeopathy, herbs, essences, etc.
2. *An Intermediate Course in Homoeopathy*. For Mum's and Dad's, to teach the next level of homoeopathic prescribing for simple conditions at home.
3. *Certificate in Homeopathic Case Taking*. To extend practical prescribing skills learnt in course 2.
4. *Practitioner Certificate in Homeopathy*. For practitioners in other modalities who want practical training in the conceptual basics of homeopathy and practical prescribing.
For details write to P.O. Box 695 Gisborne. 3437.
(03) 5427 0880. Email: admin@homstudy.net.

Other resources:
Homoeopathic remedies may be obtained from
Martin & Pleasance, 7 Rocklea Drive, Port Melbourne VIC 3207. Ph (03) 9427 7422.   **Phone and mail orders welcome.**

www.ingramcontent.com/pod-product-compliance
Lightning Source LLC
Chambersburg PA
CBHW070624290526
45790CB00002B/979